Be My Friend Until I Die:
On caring for my dying husband who has Alzheimer's

Elizabeth S Cole, MSW

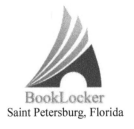

BookLocker
Saint Petersburg, Florida

Published by BookLocker.com, Inc., St. Petersburg, Florida.

Printed on acid-free paper.

BookLocker.com, Inc.
2021

First Edition

DISCLAIMER

This book details the author's personal experiences as a wife caring at home for her dying husband and about how his Alzheimer's disease shaped this care. The author is not a healthcare provider.

The author and publisher are providing this book and its contents on an "as is" basis and make no representations or warranties of any kind with respect to this book or its contents. The author and publisher disclaim all such representations and warranties, including for example warranties of merchantability and healthcare for a particular purpose. In addition, the author and publisher do not represent or warrant that the information accessible via this book is accurate, complete or current.

The statements made about products and services have not been evaluated by the U.S. Food and Drug Administration. They are not intended to diagnose, treat, cure, or prevent any condition or disease. Please consult with your own physician or healthcare specialist regarding the suggestions and recommendations made in this book.

Except as specifically stated in this book, neither the author or publisher, nor any authors, contributors, or other representatives will be liable for damages arising out of or in connection with the use of this book. This is a comprehensive limitation of liability that applies to all damages of any kind, including (without limitation) compensatory; direct, indirect or consequential damages; loss of data, income or profit; loss of or damage to property and claims of third parties.

You understand that this book is not intended as a substitute for consultation with a licensed healthcare practitioner, such as your physician. Before you begin any healthcare program, or change your lifestyle in any way, you will consult your physician or other licensed healthcare practitioner to ensure that you are in good health and that the examples contained in this book will not harm you.

This book provides content related to topics physical and/or mental health issues. As such, use of this book implies your acceptance of this disclaimer.

Dedication

John Marshall Cole (Jack) you
will be my friend forever.

Table of Contents

I was 78 and my husband 88 in 2015 when a hospice service came into our home for the first time. I had slowly become Jack's caretaker over the two years before then because of his increasing Alzheimer's disease. His moderate deafness compounded everything. Now after surgery for colon and liver cancer we were told he had not much longer to live. Jack fooled us all. After six months he got stronger and failed hospice. I think this is one of the only failures in life you really welcome.

But in the Spring of 2017, he became very sick again. This time there could be no operation. We began hospice services again. This time with Chandler Hall.

Over these years I learned every day, with many mistakes, what worked for us and what did not. I'm sharing this experience hoping that some of it may be helpful to others.

PATIENCE

It takes patience to take care of someone whose memory does not work and is still ambulatory. He gets himself food which sometimes winds up in his pockets and he puts things back where they don't belong. Frozen things wind up in the pantry and peanut butter in the freezer. He needs the same kind of supervision a five-year-old does. My Jack has liver cancer and receives hospice services. Three months ago he was given an undefined "not long to live, maybe six months". I am thankful he is in no pain. Jack eats very little and sleeps most of the day. He can get himself to the bathroom and back. I do not see the illness I expected to see in a man who may have only months to live.

Coping with this requires a different kind of patience. There is the familiar kind of patience used when you clean up the mess when something is broken. It takes another more difficult kind of patience to let the disease take its own course. There is no manual for how he will die. His course is his own. No doctor or hospice nurse, as skilled as they are, can draw a map for us. Accepting that this is, and will be, an uncharted journey is very hard. It is impossible to explain this feeling to others because I don't want him to die soon. All my life the hardest thing for me to do is to cope with the unknown. I know I can handle a short race, but can I do a marathon?

Even when I think I know how to deal with some of his behavior, it changes. It helps when I learn how to deal with some things he does. It gives me confidence that if that thing comes up again, I will know how to deal with it. Jack remembers taking pills every day. When he started hospice all these drugs were stopped. Out of the blue he asked one day for his medicine. I knew I couldn't explain why he was no longer taking pills in a way that he would understand and accept. I decided to give him a vitamin pill and say this was it. I thought the vitamin might actually help since he eats so little. This satisfies him.

It doesn't pay to get too confident because before you know it, something else quite new and different comes up. My first reaction often is, "Oh my God! What do I do now?" Once over the shock and fear I try to figure it out. The first thing I try is seldom the best solution. You learn you just have to try different things. My friend Mary Lou told me a story about when her granddaughter Ava was three. When Mary Lou got frustrated trying to put together some toy she had brought, Ava said, "Ammy, you have got to learn how to problem solve." All caretakers are problem solvers who are constantly being tested. I am learning that I may fail again and again before I find something that works. This is such a difficult lesson for us overachievers. It is humbling.

KEEPING HIS DIGNITY

Being sick is humiliating for everyone. Strangers have access to every body part and ask you to respond to embarrassing questions about bodily functions. Losing his memory has been painful for my Jack. This is a man who without a college degree holds twelve patents on manufacturing processes and products. He had so many interests. Chamber music was his favorite especially Beethoven's Late Quartets. He quoted poetry by the yard. He wrote a poem about his war experience which was published. He devoured books and loved to debate current events. Now I had to find some way to get him to wear Depends and sleep in a hospital bed. I rely on my most successful technique – I lie.

We live surrounded by woods and meadows. He loves it here. There is a bank of floor to ceiling windows in our living room overlooking our deck with flowerpots and the lawn where we have planted a tree every anniversary. I have Jack's hospital bed set up in front of the windows. He can see sky, birds, trees and flowers, and he can see who is coming up our deck to see us. He can hear his beloved music on our stereo and me puttering around in the kitchen. I learned this from my friend Velia. When her husband John was dying she had his bed set up in the living room in the middle of everything. People came and went and their dog stayed near him. She wanted whatever life he had left to be as close to normal as possible and so did I. I like the prayer, "Let me not die while I am still alive." This is my goal for my Jack, may he live as fully as he can every day he has left and not just exist.

We were fortunate because forty years ago my plan-ahead husband had a full bathroom with a walk-in shower installed off the living room for "when we got old and couldn't do the stairs". He doesn't think he is sick and asked, "Why the bed?" We have a sofa bed facing the window where I planned to sleep. I told Jack I had a really weak knee and the doctor did not want me to go up and down the stairs. I told him I didn't want to be alone and asked him if he would stay with me. Loving husband that he is, he agreed.

Explaining all the medical people coming to our house was the first big lie. Jack's medication was provided by the Veteran's Administration. We went to one of their physicians twice a year to authorize the drugs. I told him that since he was 90 he no longer had to go to the VA. They were sending nurses to him. He asked Nurse Sue if she was being paid by the federal government. She is - Medicare.

Two years ago, he learned that his cancer was untreatable and would most likely be the cause of his death. He told the oncologist that he had been an 18-year-old Marine in the South Pacific during World War II and had survived Iwo Jima. He had seen more dead people than the doctor would in his entire career. He was philosophical. He told the doctor that when he was 18 he didn't think he would live to see 19. Every day after that was a gift. He says he has had a good life and no regrets. He accepts his illness. He has no fear of death but he wants to live. Because of his last diagnosis, nothing between us and others he loves is left unsaid. What breaks my heart is when he tells me he is getting stronger every day. I smile, nod, and bite my lip to keep from sobbing.

Jack is puzzled why people come to the house when I go out. He thinks he is not very sick and is capable of caring for himself. At 90, it is insulting to have a caretaker or minder. My brilliant mechanical engineer has never learned to deal with household electronics. I am our family's electrical engineer. When caretakers come I explain that they are here to watch the house systems, the phones, the air conditioning, the Nest, and the alarm system.

Early on in his dementia I did not handle some things very well and we both suffered. I failed to remember and use something I had learned early on in my social work professional education. In my first year of graduate school I worked with two groups of children who were intellectually impaired. One group had mild to moderate deficits, the other's loss was profound. The group with the most suffering and anger was the mild to moderate group. They knew there was something wrong with them. They were different and were sensitive about it. They blew up at me when I offered the slightest correction. When Jack's memory was failing I would question his recollection of events if they were way off. This made him very angry. For example, he told me that early in our marriage I had moved to California and lived there seventeen years. When I protested that this never happened he got very angry at me and I at him for not accepting what was the truth. I was hurt. Was this his way to tell me that I had let him down? I would dissect his words like I was analyzing a poem for hidden meanings. This was not working for us. But the lie did. The next time he told me this I apologized to him and asked for forgiveness saying, "I was young and foolish." The issue was dropped and forgotten. What I learned is that correcting someone who has dementia is not a winning game. You may be correct but the more important question to ask yourself is, "What do I win if I win?" I now agree with everything he says except anything that would harm him or me.

Listening to what he says with love is a gift I try to give him every day. So much of what he says doesn't make much sense or it is repetitive. I also learned from my challenged clients that while they may not always understand what you say to them, they frequently sense what you feel about them. This wasn't too hard for me; it was reminiscent of the way I didn't understand a word when Jack tried to explain to me what string theory was in mathematics. I didn't have to feign the love.

One of my tasks has been sparing him sorrow. Lately he has wanted to see his mother who has been long gone. He misses her and wants us to pick her up and bring her for dinner. He thinks she might be living in our barn. Early on when he asked about his mother I told him she had died. Now I know that it is not helpful. It makes him sad. I tell him she has gone to Nova Scotia to paint. He vaguely remembers her going there in the past. He also asks about his older brother, Ed. I tell Jack that Ed is in France with his French wife Gabriele. He asks me that several times a day. Jack's sister Muriel died last week. I will not tell him.

I lie a lot about money. My Jack was a child of the depression. Although his father had a job as a school teacher, sometimes the milk bill for his five children didn't get paid on time. Jack now thinks things cost the same as they did in the 30s and 40s. He is shocked when a sandwich costs $10. I say it is for two or more. I have learned the hard way that I have to warn service people who come to the house what to tell him their services cost. I had hired two young men to come with their chain saws to cut up some trees that had fallen in our meadow. When they came, I was taking a shower. Jack told them we would give them $5 an hour and they left.

IT TAKES A VILLAGE (BUT YOU MIGHT NOT ALWAYS WANT IT)

We are fortunate because we have support. The Chandler Hall hospice team is a comforting convoy on this journey. Sue, Jessica, Cindy, and Chris support me at every turn. We are able to hire aides from Seniors Helping Seniors of Bucks County so that I can get out. My friends and family are willing to help any way they can. I have learned that some help is not very helpful and that I sometimes stand in the way of help.

When people learn of Jack's sickness they all express a willingness to help. I just had to call them and tell them what I needed, and they would be there. Yet here I am after 35 years as a social worker, a helping professional, finding it so hard to ask for, and accept help. Am I an overachiever? Yes! Do I think I can do this myself?

I start thinking of how I feel when I help friends. It feels good to help my 93-year-old neighbor Mabel by visiting and bringing lunch. I liked the way I felt about myself when I transported a friend in a nursing home to our book club. I suspect that those who help me would feel the same way. I am just beginning to reach out. I have begun making a specific list of how I would like to be helped. Friends offer to go out to lunch with me. I have asked them to bring lunch to me. We can sit on my deck and be as leisurely as we want. I don't have to look at my watch and worry if I have to get home so the aide can leave. Besides, a bonus is that Jack sometimes joins us and likes hearing the voices and laughter. My sister Sue is a terrific soup maker. I will ask her to make me some once a month. Jack loves soup. It is one of the few things he will eat. Food is a good way to help. Having fewer meals to plan, shop for and prepare is a help. I can drive, but having someone drive me places is an energy saver and I feel pampered.

My niece Regan has been great help to me and to her uncle. Her caring for him shows through whatever she does for the both of us. She is helping me do all the things I wanted to do around the house but cannot find the time or energy to do.

While failing to use the help offered is difficult, harder yet is to defend against unwanted help. Some of it feels like assault. Assault with a friendly weapon – but no less assault. I believe we judge people by what we believe is right and wrong. We measure the actions of others by whether we would do the same thing in their circumstances. When we see others making "mistakes" that may not be helpful to themselves or others, we sometimes offer "helpful advice". What has been hard for me is that some well-intentioned people are sure that they know what I should be doing for my Jack and for me and it is not what I am doing. I want to keep him home. He loves it here. He so appreciates the sky, trees, flowers and wildlife. One suggestion was that I put him upstairs in our bedroom. That way I would have "the downstairs for myself without all the disruption". Others genuinely worry that this care will be too hard for me. And that I should place him in a nursing home. Caring for him could injure my health. "You have no life and at your age every day is precious." They argue that this 90-year-old man who sometimes does not remember who I am "is not the love of my younger years. He is gone." One day he did say, "I sometimes do not know who you are, but I know what you are."

I cannot do this. I have spent most of my adult life loving him. Though faded, those are the blue eyes I always found attractive. I come from a family where my grandparents and my mother were cared for at home. Leaving him would not be me. I also recognize that others may not have had this choice and that one day circumstances may make placing him a necessity for me. While I know deep down that these people really do want to help, I have to confess, it makes me angry. Implied in all this is criticism that I am making bad choices. Unless you have been a caretaker, you cannot appreciate how painful this is because we judge ourselves constantly and find ourselves wanting most of the time. We worry over every decision. Is this the right one?

My social worker Jess has been a great help to me in sorting out how I feel and what I truly want to do.

WHAT HAS HELPED?

What has helped is people staying in touch by calling and emailing me regularly. I can feel their affection and it is soothing. A dear friend in Scotland calls regularly.

My friend Carol is a constant source of support and good advice. This is based not only on her experience as a skilled family therapist, but the time she spent caring for her late husband whose condition mirrored Jack's.

Find some humor in daily life. Recently Jack told me that we had a communication problem because we are from two different countries. He also asked who were the four people who were in bed with me. I never knew I had such an exciting and X-rated life...

He has kept a large part of his sense of humor. Today Nurse Sue and I were looking at a photograph of him taken 15 years ago. He asked me who that man was. I said he was the love of my life. He replied, "Well, you could have done better."

Yesterday when I came in from shopping, Nurse Sue said, "Here comes your wife." He said, "It is she who must be obeyed," the nickname he had for me from watching the TV series Rumpole of the Bailey.

Sunday was a quiet day after a week of visitors and caretakers. Jack asked me, "Where is our staff?" I told him it was Sunday and they had the day off.

I really like when someone invites me to do something they plan. My friend Barbara knows I love opera. She finds out when the Metropolitan Opera's encore performance is playing in a nearby theater. She comes with her husband Bud who stays with Jack and Barb takes me to the opera. It helps not having to plan everything and have someone take you. I feel pampered. I think I need more of this.

One morning my husband said, "It has been a pleasure knowing you." He always thanks me for what I do for him and asks me what he can do for me. There are sweet moments like this and many peaceful days. If I am honest with myself, I recognize that caretaking is not a role that you enjoy much of the time. It is hard work.

You often feel frustrated, angry, deprived, and depressed. I sometimes want to run away from it all. Chasing right behind all of these feelings is strong guilt. You should not be feeling this way. This is the man you have loved for forty-nine years. You choose this.

I believe that we cannot control feelings. They just come. We are responsible for what we do about them. This is not easy. I cannot confess how strong these feelings are to everyone, especially those who do not think I should be caring for him. This isolates me from some people. My mantra has become, "You are not a saint." This gets repeated frequently. Of course, if you want this reinforced, speak to one of your siblings. They know fully well from your childhood that you are not a saint. I can and do talk to my family and best friends. It helps a lot. They offer me absolution.

It is hard for caregivers to forgive themselves. My psychologist friend Bridget said it helps if you have some "nails" to "hang" your anger on. This week I am angry that the Phillies don't play better than they do... and why does packaging have to be as hard as it is to open? Our current political scene can provide unlimited "nails" regardless of your point of view.

This makes me think how much harder all this must be for caretakers who do not love the family member they are helping. There are those who receive no thanks and just anger for what they do. This is truly a work of mercy. As hard as it is, it has got to be much easier to take care of someone you love and like rather than someone you don't, or someone who has never really liked you.

My 93year-old friend Mabel has a sign on her computer that says, "What have you done today to make yourself happy?" This squares with my belief that you are responsible for your own happiness. Other people can be sources of happiness for you, and may want to make you happy but they are not responsible for your happiness – you are. What do I do?

I love classical music. It is so evocative. I cannot listen to Bach, Mozart, or Handel without feeling good. I love opera. Some arias make my heart soar; others mirror my sadness. Celtic music makes me want to dance. My sister Sue, also a Bach lover, likes to dance around her kitchen to Joe Cocker. My radio is tuned to classic music much of the day.

A cup of Prince of Wales tea and a good mystery are soothing. So is a British series on TV.

I try not to miss my monthly mystery book club meeting at the New Hope Library and my bimonthly neighborhood book club.

My friend Carol gave me a birthday gift of a ticket to see *Hello Dolly* with Bette Midler in NYC. Her son-in-law David and his wife Jill drove us into the city. Pure joy for three hours. I was able to relax because I had two shifts of private duty nurses with hospice experience staying with Jack.

Caretaking makes you super conscious of time passing. All my working life I ran from task to task. I am trying to slow down and savor more. I am learning from Jack who revels at the shades of green in our trees or the patterns in the clouds. I need help in knowing how to do this.

I have been intrigued with the concept of mindfulness – being focused and present in a non-judgmental way with what is happening in the moment. I have just begun reading about it.

Yesterday I listened to a guided meditation to help me relax. The first 45-minute exercise promoted deep relaxation. At the end of the time I felt really tired. Later as I grocery shopped I almost wept. I thought I should be feeling better. What I think happened is that the deep relaxation took the lid off some exhaustion that I have been tamping down for a long time. Perhaps it helped to release some devils. We will see.

Seeing Summer and Claudia my granddaughters" names on caller ID makes me smile in anticipation.

My tranquilizer of choice is chocolate.

My step-daughter Karen and her husband Rick try to come down from Connecticut as often as they can. She wants me to go away at least one weekend a month. I don't have the desire or energy to take a trip. So I go to the Manion Ranch (my cheaper version of the Canyon Ranch), my sister Sue's house 15 miles away where I get pampered and, bless heaven, left alone.

Karen calls twice a day on her way to and from work.

People pray for me and Jack and I am grateful. I too pray. Mine are mostly pleas for help or of thanksgiving when I realize how lucky I am that he is not suffering, that we have support, and that we have had each other for so long.

I do believe knowledge is power. Studying about what I am facing has always helped me feel better armed to deal with it. Jack was diagnosed with Alzheimer's after a CT scan and six hours of psychometric testing. His neurologist and the psychologist were very thorough. They went over all the test results. We could see that Jack's brain had shrunken a bit. The scan let us look down on his brain. There were black dots scattered on the surface. This is the amyloid plaque. I think of this picture when I realize that there are portions of his brain which seemed untouched. He still has a quick wit. I used to think that dementia was like a glass of water with the level slowly but uniformly going down. I am now convinced it is more like Swiss cheese where portions remain relatively unscathed for a long time. The neurologist was thorough in explaining the nature of the condition and the usual course it takes. The psychologist pointed out that Jack was a visual learner and was in the 95th percentile of people who retain what they read. This was a key diagnostic find because it leads me to realize that I should write things down rather than tell him things.

I was helped with the medical language in the reports about his liver cancer by my granddaughter Claudia, and my brother-in-law and sister-in-law, Paul and Arlene, all nurse practitioners. It really does help to have a translator. I know our hospice nurse would also help with this. Knowing we can contact our doctor friend Mahshid is also a comfort. The oncologist said Jack's liver cancer had dramatically increased and could not be cured. We were referred that day to the Chandler Hall hospice.

Months ago, I decided I wanted to try an educational lecture designed specifically for new caretakers. I was looking forward to getting some tips. My sister Mary Ellen went with me to a meeting at a memory care facility. The room was packed. The speaker was introduced. She had lots of experience in dealing with people with Alzheimer's from caring for her own family members to her professional experiences. The speech had good information. The question and answer period was not helpful. While she had lots to share, she was not an experienced group leader. The audience was desperate for help. One or two monopolized the time and she didn't know how to stop them. The group became restive. It was not a good experience. As we were filing out of the room, the marketing director said, "Remember, 80% of all caregivers die before the person with dementia." We left with that cheery ending. Note to self, pick group meetings more carefully.

While I focus on each day as it comes, it is helpful to plan for what comes next. What will I do when Jack's condition is such that it will not be appropriate to leave him with the paid aides or family members? What will happen when his physical care is too hard for me? I had to deal with that when I went into NYC for the day. It was too long to leave him with amateur or volunteer aides. Hospice helped me locate two retired hospice nurses who do private duty work. They came so I could relax and enjoy.

It is painful but I have begun to plan for the worst before I am at my worst. I now have an outline for funeral services for Jack. I want people to know him from the eyes of those who knew him: Karen knew him as the single father who raised her, my granddaughters as their grandfather, his brother Paul and his niece Barbara who has spent lots of time with him.

A friend, a recent widow, wished they had had more time to work on an obituary. I plan to ask my writer brother-in-law Jim to do it.

The first time Jack was in hospice in 2015, he was with a different provider. I met their social worker during that period, and about ten minutes after she came into our house, she asked Jack and me if we had planned for the funeral and handed us some materials.

The social work supervisor in me almost hit the roof. She knew nothing about us, or if we had discussed death and dying, much less a funeral. Somebody needed more training. When I got to know her better, I told her that what she had done was not helpful and why. It was probably less painful for Jack and me than lots of others because we have always discussed what we would like, and our Karen knows our wishes. Afterwards, I did visit a funeral parlor. Jack wishes to be cremated. The staff person gave me a catalogue of containers for his ashes. Most were very costly and very ugly. When he noticed my dismay, the young director said, "Of course you may use any container you wish. Is there anything he loves?" There is. Our Seattle friend Betty gave him a blue glazed pot with a lid made by her favorite Japanese potter. I got to thinking about what I would want. I think the red Italian Amaretti can will suit me just fine.

TAKING CARE OF ME

While many things sooth my spirit, it has proven difficult for me to be conscientious about my health. I have Psoriasis and Diabetes. Psoriasis is an annoyance. I have been through all the treatments and know that it comes and goes and may flare with stress.

Diabetes is harder in many ways. It silently injures. When my skin itches or feels like a brush burn, it is a signal that I have to do something about it to make it stop. There are few symptoms from diabetes until it is left uncontrolled. It can sometimes damage your organs beyond repair. It is time consuming. There are doctors to see beyond my internist; ophthalmologists, periodontists, podiatrists. Blood has to be tested several times a day and taken at a lab quarterly. Medications are taken twice and an insulin injection every night. There is a certain tyranny to the care. I found this hard to do before becoming a caretaker and could easily find excuses to ignore being rigorous. Caretaking, if I let it, could be a big cop out for not doing all that I should be doing. I have to guard against this. I have created reminders. My friend Carol calls me regularly, and every time she does she asks if I have been testing, and what my blood sugar is. My Amazon Echo Alexa is like Siri on steroids. I ask her to remind me every day to take my medicine and every night if I have taken my insulin.

Sleep has always been a great curative for me. For the last few weeks I haven't gotten much because Jack is restless and frequently gets up to go to the bathroom. Last night he filled the sink to wash his hands and left the water running in the stoppered sink. I caught it in time. He has forgotten how to cover himself with his blanket. Since he is always cold I need to tuck him in after each trip. I have safeguards against him getting out of the house. One door to the outside has a lock that gets stuck and takes a lot of noisy effort to open. I have put sleigh bells on the other door so I can hear it opening. Nurse Sue recommends that I give him a mild sedative at bed time.

I hope that works, I need sleep. If it doesn't, I may take the sedative.

It did not work. Next week a nurse I hired will stay with him Wednesday night so I can get some sleep. Nurse Liza has come into our lives. She comes every Wednesday night at 9pm. She stays so I can sleep in my own bed through the night. I am grateful.

THE LAST FEW MONTHS

September

This is where I am now this first week of September 2017. It will be interesting to see how things change with time. Jack has begun to complain of pressure in his side where his liver is when he sits or stands for any length of time. He is most comfortable stretched out in bed. He sleeps most of the day, eats very little, and rarely sits in his beloved recliner.

So far, all I have talked about is the stress of being a caretaker. I am a wife, but I am also a stepmother, a mother-in-law, a grandmother, a sister, an aunt and a friend. I am blessed by the closeness I have with those I love. These ties also bring worry. Right now, I am anxious to hear how my sister Adrienne rode out the hurricane in Florida. None of my sisters are free from illness. One of my sisters has a serious chronic illness. Every time I see her I look to see how she is handling the fatigue it brings. What worries those I love worries me. My friend Mary Lou counsels, "Try to worry only about the things you can control." This is very hard to do. The pain of worrying is the price we pay for love.

This morning I read my *New Hope Newsletter*. It is filled with all of the wonderful places to go and all of the appealing events coming up. I wanted to do them all. When I processed that I couldn't because I had to be here, I was filled with resentment. Then I realized I was having a "taking away my car keys moment". Someone I know, who rarely drives and almost never at night, was told she couldn't drive at night because of an eye condition. She was angry. "Now what will I do?" We both laughed when I pointed out that she hadn't driven at night for years, and probably wouldn't have *even if* the Department of Motor Vehicle people *hadn't told her she couldn't*. What she didn't like was the thought that she couldn't if she wanted to. A bit of independence was gone even if her lifestyle hadn't changed at all. The same thing had just happened to me. Even if I wasn't a caretaker I would not have gone to most of the events I had read about. Note to me – guard against faux deprivations.

September 15

I think the other shoe has dropped. My sister Sue and my sister from another mother, Laura, brought lunch and we all sat on my sun filled deck eating the wonderful soup and salad. Jack ate with gusto all of his soup and two helpings of salad. Nurse Sue came bringing him more chicken soup. We brought him to his bed and she examined him. He complained that his ribs were pressing on something. She told me that for the first time she felt a mass and that his expanded liver was pressing on his ribs when he sat up. At this time the pain is momentary and is relieved when he is on his back. No need for painkillers yet. Nurse Sue notices that he may have an eye infection, conjunctivitis? She orders drops which he is to get every three hours he is awake.

October

Jack's clothing tells the story of his illness. Going through his closet I find jeans starting at size 40 and ending with the last pair I bought him two months ago, size 32. These are too large for him and I am now getting him sweatpants with an elastic waist and drawstring. He will never get into any of his shirts again. Even his shoes don't want to stay on his feet so I bought him those heavy duty hospital socks with ribs on the bottom. I have given some of his clothes away. I am taking the shirts to be washed and ironed before giving them away. Jess, my social worker, told me that they had a quilt made for her brother after their father died. What a great idea. Then I remembered that my niece Kate took some of her late father's shirts to a friend with a patchwork business. She had bears made of the shirts for her three children. I knew what I would do. I will have three afghans made, one for Karen, Summer and Claudia. I contacted the Quilted Bear in Princeton and got instructions on how to proceed. I am excited to see what they will look like. My sisters Sue and Mary Ellen and I make a trip to Princeton to deliver the shirts. We meet my nephew David for lunch. A good day out.

If Jack's clothing tells a story so does mine. I bought new slacks one size smaller. My doctor will be pleased.

I hug Jack every day as often as I can. Yesterday he said, "I am lazy and happy." It occurs to me again that unless men are gay, and if they do not have women or children in their lives, they do not get long hugs or prolonged touching and tenderness. I am so sorry for those who live, or are dying without this. I want to hug all the family less men in hospice. I would probably be arrested.

October 8

Coleen, the nurse practitioner, came to examine Jack. She could not feel a mass. Jack still eats little and sleeps most of the day. I wish he would sleep more at night. His hospice care was extended another two months. I am so relieved. We get so much support from the hospice team. Not a week goes by when I do not hear from or see his nurse, Sue, our social worker, Jess, or his physical therapist, Cindy.

October 11

Barbara and I go to the movie to see a taped production of the Met's *Norma*. It was wonderful. I heard a terrific soprano for the first time, Sondra Radvonofsky. Joyce DiDonato was great as usual.

October 16

I feel a weariness that no sleep, meditation or distraction will lift. My Seton Hill University motto is, "Hazard yet forward."

Some things in life must just be borne. On the table by my chair is a stack of books. The self-help ones have edged out my mysteries. These books show me how to meditate, relieve stress, and be a better caretaker. Sometimes, I think they are a burden. When there are days like today, I feel I must be doing what they say wrong because of my weariness. I now think the problem must be in my expectation. What they teach temporarily helps lift what I feel, but will never take it all away. I told my good friend Phillida how I felt. She reminded me of the advice we had received on parenting from the British psychologist, David Winnicut. He said, "Do not expect perfect parenting, look for good enough." She said this applies to caretaking as well. I think she is right.

All of this makes me think of the place pain has in all our lives. Growing up pain was accepted as normal. It was a part of life. The nuns taught us to "offer it up". My parents just carried on through it, showing us what adults do. Today I think things are different. There are hundreds of books and apps to help us avoid pain, relieve stress. Painkillers are handed out at the slightest complaint. My granddaughter was given oxycodone by her dentist when he pulled two teeth.

Perhaps as a society we now think pain is abnormal and should be denied or avoided. Suffering is a part of life as is losing the people we love. I think we would be better if we could just accept this.

The nights are getting colder. I have just ordered a down comforter for my always cold Jack. I also bought him an electric mattress pad so he will be snug. My goal is to keep him warm and secure and peaceful.

October 25

Four of my oldest friends came to my annual Halloween lunch. I have known them all for over 50 years. Some have known Jack longer than I have. He joins us for lunch and eats more than he has for a week. I think it is the socialization. He isn't aware he is eating. Maybe tomorrow I will bring people in off the road with a "free meals sign" so Jack will have an appetite.

There are times I know caring for him here is worth it. One day I asked him what I could do for him. He said, "Take care of yourself and be my friend until I die."

He is not lucid most of the time, except every morning when he wakes up, he says, "How beautiful this is. Look at the trees and the sky." He loves a first thing glass of orange juice and never fails to say, "This is so good." He is alive, not just existing. He always thanks me every time I do something for him.

November

November 3

There is a change in Jack's behavior. He has become more agitated. There is a qualitative difference to his wandering mind. It is hard to describe. It seems more hallucinogenic. He seems less anchored to reality and he is testy and snaps at everyone. At one point he says to me, "Who do you think you are, God?" I go into another room and cry. I don't know how much longer I can take this. This is so hard. When I come back to see him, he has forgotten that he was angry with me. On one level I know it is his dementia that was talking, but it still hurts. My night nurse Liza says that sometimes when the kidneys break down ammonia and other chemicals in the blood are not eliminated. They circulate and affect the brain. She cautioned that if Karen wanted to spend time with her father she should come now.

November 5

Nurse Sue visits. Jack is irritable and insists we must leave now to shop for bread, milk and cheese for the "children who are hungry". After Sue leaves, Jack goes into the bathroom, thinking the door to the outside is there. He insists that we must go out for food. He is angry when I tell him that we cannot. He says, "I want to go home!" I tell him I will take him home and I lead him back to bed. Exhausted, he sleeps. I become more alert at night fearing he will get out of bed and wander. The agitation lasts all weekend. Nurse Sue came Monday, Jess, the social worker came on Tuesday. I speak to Cindy, his physical therapist. We talk about what could possibly be done to support me in caring for Jack.

November 8

Independent Jack still gets out of bed and tries to get to the bathroom. He falls. I am not strong enough to pick him up and I have to call the EMS. Our local policemen come and take him back to bed.

November 9-10

During the night his feet slide out of bed towards the floor. I try to get him to put them back. He either can't, or won't. I pick up his legs several times during the night. It is hard. I do not think of myself as a weak person but I realize that I am not strong enough. I am awake most of the night. That day Jess and Cindy and Sue come out to see Jack. Sue gives him medication meant to calm him down. I had called Karen and Rick and they were there from Connecticut. When Jack first started with his hospice team, I spoke to them about something I wanted them to do for me. I told them that I am a "never say die" person and might try to care for Jack after I am able to. Jess had told me that there will be a time when I must step back and just be his wife.

He needs more care than I can give him. They arrange for him to go into hospice at Chandler Hall. Meanwhile he is given morphine and something for the agitation.

At 7pm an ambulance came. I went with Jack in the ambulance while Karen and Rick followed behind. Jack thanked the EMS men for their kindness. In his all mixed up mind there are these moments of lucidity. My heart wrenches when I realize this might have been the last time we were in our house together.

I am now going to sound like a commercial for Chandler Hall. By now you know how highly I think of the team who came to my house. We felt just as welcomed by the staff in the residence. They are kind and caring and make us feel that there isn't anything they wouldn't do for Jack and us. There is a level of caring I never felt during his last hospice experience.

Jack has been an anomaly. No one can figure out how he has continued to be so strong because he eats so little and is so thin. We are told that while there is no way they can predict the day of his death, we should tell anyone who wants to say goodbye to come now. They think that while it may not be days, it will not be weeks.

When we get home we begin to notify his family and plan for his funeral. In the middle of talking calmly and being efficient, we sob. Karen and Rick go back to Connecticut to take care of work obligations. I cannot sleep. I follow the same caretaker schedule – up every two hours.

November 11

Sunday, my sister Mary Ellen comes to take me to see Jack. She brings the quilts I had made from Jack's shirts for Karen, Claudia, and Summer. They are beautiful. When we get to Chandler we find Nurse Sue, who was visiting him on her day off. I am not sure Jack knows I am there. When I hold his hand and say I love you, he says it back. I soon run out of gas and am taken home so I can get to bed. It takes a while because, lucky me, I get calls from so many friends offering love and support. I confess (Dr. Shonberg, don't read this) that my dinner was left over mashed potatoes, green beans, and Swiss almond chocolate ice cream. Nary a protein in sight.

November 12

When I call this morning, I am told that Jack had a restless night. He got out of bed to go to the bathroom, fell, and told the nurse that I was sitting in the corner. I am comforted that he thinks I am always with him. He is off medication this morning. I spend time calling the caretakers to cancel this week's schedule. Karen and I visit. Jack has been moved to a private room across from the nurses' station. Karen goes back to Connecticut.

November 13

Regan drives me to see Jack. He is sleeping peacefully. His hands are warm for the first time in weeks. I lean over to say I love you and he mouths something back. I think it was I love you too. He always said that. When I hold his hand under the covers he grasps it hard, as though he is clinging. Cindy and Jess stop by to see us. Late afternoon I feel so tired I feel faint. Regan and I kiss Jack goodbye. He is snoring quietly,

November 14

I could not sleep at all. At 3am I gave up pretending, and came down to read a book. At 4:55am, I received a call from Chandler. Jack had died peacefully in his sleep five minutes prior. I knew this could happen at any time. Was I prepared? Oh no. Could this be true? They didn't think it would be days. Why did I come home? Maybe I should have slept in the chair by his bed so he wouldn't have been alone. I call Karen and Rick who leave to come down. She calls the girls.

November 15

The funeral director says the earliest they can arrange a funeral is November 20. Karen, Rick, and my granddaughters arrive and set everything in motion. While I had outlined the funeral service, Karen fleshed it out and notified those who were to speak. She also took over organization of the luncheon to follow the service. As a development director, she does this for a living. All is a fog to me. People bring food. Late that afternoon, Karen and I go to the funeral home to see her father. I am frightened that I won't hold up. It was so good to see him. He looked peaceful and dignified. He was my old Jack, thinner, but my old Jack.

There is a problem. The pottery container I had picked for his ashes takes up all the space in our niche. There will be no space for mine.

I instruct the funeral director to fill it half up with Jack's ashes and then to put my ashes in it when I die. He will give me what doesn't go into the urn.

November 20

The days leading up to the service have been a blur. I cannot tell you what has happened, or on what day. I know all I felt was exhaustion. The service was beautiful. It was a real tribute to my Jack by those who loved him. The funeral director told me that when he arranged the Marine Honor Guard to come to the service, he told them that Jack had been in the Battle of Iwo Jima. Eight Marines in full dress came. Seven Marines shot three volleys for a 21-gun salute and a bugler blew taps. As they folded the flag, they put the empty shell cases in it. I gave it to Karen. I already had the flags that Jack had bought and proudly hung.

November 24

All have gone. I am finally alone to grieve. I take Jack's remaining ashes and spread them under all the trees we had bought for our wedding anniversaries and I cried. It was the farewell I had wanted and didn't get at the formal service. I shall miss my love's physical presence but his memory will always be with me. I was so blessed to have him in my life.

CPSIA information can be obtained
at www.ICGtesting.com
Printed in the USA
BVHW070050080321
601925BV00006B/9